Relation of the Mineral Salts of the Body to the Signs of the Zodiac

DR. GEORGE W. CAREY

Price, 25c

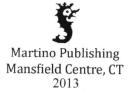

Martino Publishing
Mansfield Centre, CT
2013

Martino Publishing
P.O. Box 373,
Mansfield Centre, CT 06250 USA

ISBN 978-1-61427-421-6

© *2013 Martino Publishing*

Cover design by T. Matarazzo

Printed in the United States of America On 100% Acid-Free Paper

Relation of the
Mineral Salts of the Body
to the
Signs of the Zodiac

Price, 25c

DR. GEORGE W. CAREY

BIOCHEMISTRY

Acid and Alkali acting,
Proceeding and acting again.
Operating, transmuting, fomenting
In throes and spasms of pain—
Uniting, reacting, creating,
Like souls "passing under the rod"—
Some people call it Chemistry,
And others call it God.

Biochemistry means that Chemistry of Life, or the union of inorganic and organic substances whereby new compounds are formed.

In its relation to so-called disease this system uses the inorganic salts, known as Cell-Salts, or tissue builders.

The constituent parts of man's body are perfect principles, namely, oxygen, hydrogen, carbon, lime, iron, potash, soda, silica, magnesia, etc. These elements, gases, etc., are perfect per se, but may be endlessly diversified in combination as may the planks, bricks or stones with which a building is to be erected.

A shadow cannot be removed by chemicals; neither can disease be removed by poison. There is nothing (no thing) to be removed in either case; but there is a deficiency to be supplied. The shadow may be removed by supplying light to the space covered by the shadow.

So symptoms, called disease, disappear or cease to manifest when the food called for is furnished.

The human body is a receptacle for a storage battery, and will always run right while the chemicals are present in proper quantity and combination, as surely as an automobile will run when charged and supplied with the necessary ingredients to vibrate or cause motion.

The cell-salts are found in all our food, and are thus carried into the blood, where they carry on the process of life, and by the law of Chemical Affinity keep the human form, bodily functions, materialized. When a deficiency occurs in any of these workers through a non-assimilation of food, poor action of liver or digestive process, dematerialization of the body commences. So disease is a deficiency in some of the chemical constituents that carry on the chemistry of life, and not an entity.

Having learned that disease is not a thing, but a condition due to lack of some inorganic constituent of the blood, it follows naturally that the proper method of cure is to supply the blood with that which is lacking. In the treatment of disease the use of anything not a constituent of the blood is unnecessary.

Dr. Chas. W. Littlefield, Analytical Chemist, says:

"The twelve mineral salts are, in a very real sense, the material basis of the organs and tissues of the body and are absolutely essential to their integrity of structure and functional activity. Experiments prove that the various tissue cells will rapidly disintegrate in the absence of the proper proportion of these salts in the circulating fluid. Whereas the maintenance

of this proportion insures healthy growth and perpetual renewal.
"These mineral salts are, therefore, the physical basis of all
healing. Regardless of the school employed, if these are absent
from the blood and tissues, no permanent cure is possible."

Osteopathy, mechano-therapy, Chiropractic, electro-therapy, naturopathy, hydropathy, massage, suggestion, mental healing, magnetic healing, etc., are all advanced agents in keeping the human organism in perfect poise. But, first of all methods, comes Biochemistry to supply deficiencies in the blood. "The blood is the life," and without perfect blood, health is impossible.

ESOTERIC CHEMISTRY

In this strenuous age of reconstruction, while God's creative compounds are forming a new race in the morning of a new age, all who desire physical regeneration should strive by every means within their reach to build a new tissue, nerve fluids and brain cells, thus literally making "new bottles for the new wine." For be it known to all men that the word "wine" as used in Scripture, means blood when used in connection with man. It also means the sap of trees and juice of vegetables or fruit.

The parable of turning water into wine at the marriage of Cana in Galilee is a literal statement of a process taking place every heart beat in the human organism.

Galilee means a circle of water or fluid—the circulatory system. Cana means a dividing place—the lungs. In the Greek, "A place of reeds," or cells of lungs that vibrate sound.

Biochemists have shown that food does not form blood, but simply furnishes the mineral base by setting free the inorganic or cell-salts contained in all food stuff. The organic part, oil, fibrin, albumen, etc., contained in food is burned or digested in the stomach and intestinal tract to furnish motive power to operate the human machine and draw air into lungs, thence into arteries, i.e., air carriers.

Therefore, it is clearly proven that air (spirit) unites with the minerals and forms blood, proving that the oil, albumen, etc., found in blood, is created every breath at the "marriage in Cana of Galilee."

Air was called water or the pure sea, viz.: Virgin Mar-y. So we see how water is changed into wine—blood—every moment.

In the new age, we will need perfect bodies to correspond with the higher vibration, or motion of the new blood, for "old bottles (bodies) cannot contain the new wine."

Another allegorical statement typifying the same truth reads, "And I saw a new Heaven and a new Earth," i.e., a new mind and new body.

Biochemistry may well say with Walt Whitman: "To the sick lying on their backs I bring help, and to the strong, upright man I bring more needed help." To be grouchy, cross, irritable, despondent or easily discouraged, is prima facie evidence that the fluids of the stomach, liver and brain are not vibrating at normal rate, the rate that results in equilibrium or health. Health cannot be qualified, i.e., poor health or good health. There must be either health or dishealth; ease or disease. We do not say poor ease or good ease. We say ease or disease, viz., not at ease.

A sufficient amount of the cell-salts of the body, properly combined and taken as food— not simply to cure some ache, pain or exudation—forms blood that materializes in healthy fluids, flesh and bone tissue.

We should take the tissue cell-salts as one uses health foods, not simply to change not health to health, but to keep the rate of blood vibration in the tone of health all the time.

THE ULTIMATE OF BIOCHEMISTRY

The microscope increases the rate of motion of the cells of the retina and we see things that were occulted to the natural rate of vibration of sight cells. Increase the rate of activity of brain cells by supplying more of the dynamic molecules of the blood known as mineral or cell-salts of lime, potash, sodium, iron, magnesia, silica, and we see mentally, truths that we could not sense at lower or natural rates of motion, although the lower rate may manifest ordinary health.

Natural man, or natural things, must be raised from the level of nature to super-natural, in order to realize new concepts that lie waiting for recognition above the solar-plexus, that is, above the animal or natural man.

The positive pole of Being must be "lifted

up" from the Kingdom of Earth, animal desire below the solar-plexus, to the pineal gland which connects the cerebellum, the temple of the Spiritual Ego, with the optic thalmus, the third eye.

By this regenerative process millions of dormant cells of the brain are resurrected and set in operation, and then man no longer "sees through a glass darkly," but with the Eye of Spiritual understanding.

To those who object to linking chemistry with astrology, the writer has this to say:

The Cosmic Law is not in the least disturbed by negative statements of the ignorant individual. Those investigators of natural phenomena, who delve deeply to find Truth, pay little heed to the babbler who says, "I can't understand how the zodiacal signs can have any relation to the cell-salts of the human body." The sole reason that he "cannot understand" is because he never tried to understand.

A little earnest, patient study will open the understanding of any one possessed of ordinary intelligence and make plain the great truth that the UNIverse is what the word implies, i.e., **one verse.**

It logically follows that all parts of one thing are susceptible to the operation of any part.

The human body is an epitome of the cosmos.

Each sign of the Zodiac is represented by the twelve functions of the body and the position of the Sun at birth.

Therefore the cell-salt coreresponding with the Sign of the Zodiac and function of the body is consumed more rapidly than other salts and needs an extra amount to supply the deficiency caused by the Sun's influence at that particular time.

Space will only permit a brief statement of the awakening of humanity to great occult truths. However, the following from India will indicate the trend of new thought: "Dr. Carey's remarkable researches in the domain of healing art have left no stone unturned. His discovery of the Zodiacal cell-salts has added a new page in the genesis of healing art," writes Swaminatha Bomiah, M. B., Ph. D. Sc., F. I. A. C., in an article in Self-Culture Magazine, published at No. 105 Armenian St., G. T., Madras, India.

THE TWELVE CELL SALTS OF THE ZODIAC

* * *

ARIES: "THE LAMB OF GOD"
March 21 to April 19

Astrologers have for many years waited for the coming discovery of a planet to rule the head or brain of man, symbolized in the "Grand Man" of the heavens by the celestial sign of the zodiac, regnant from March 21st to April 19. This sign is known as Aries—the Ram or Lamb.

Angles of planets cause effects or influences. The Priesthood of the middle ages, wishing to control the ignorant masses, personified the influence of planetary aspects, positions or angles, and transposed the letters so they spelled Angel. Upon this one "slippery cog" the stupendous frauds of Ecclesiasticism were built.

With the false teachings of the Church ingrained into the fibre of the brain of man, is it strange that for years before the advent of a new planet, with its added angle (influence), that the brain cells of Earth's inhabitants should be disturbed, as the effects of the coming storms disturb the fluids and mechanism of the weather forecaster's laboratory?

The coming of Christ and the end of the world has been preached from every street corner for several years, and thousands, yea, millions, are pledging themselves to try to live as Christ lived or according to their concept of His life.

No great movement of the people ever occurs without a scientific cause.

The Optic Thalmus, meaning "light of the chamber," is the inner or third eye, situated in the center of the head. It connects the pineal gland and the pituitary body. The optic nerve starts from this "eye single." "If thine eye be single, thy whole body will be full of light." The **optic thalmus is the Aries planet** and when fully developed through physical regeneration (see Part II in "Wonders of the Human Body"), it lifts the initiate up from the Kingdom of Earth, animal desire below the solar plexus, to the pineal gland that connects the cerebellum, the temple of the Spiritual Ego, with the optic thalmus, the third eye.

By this regenerative process millions of dormant cells of the brain are resurrected and set in operation, and then man no longer "sees through a glass darkly," but with the Eye of spiritual understanding.

I venture to predict that the planet corresponding to the optic thalmus will soon be located in the heavens.

"The new order cometh."

In ancient lore Aries was known as the "Lamb of Gad," or God, which represents the head or brain. The brain controls and directs the body and mind of man. The brain itself, however, is a receiver operated upon by celestial influences or angles (angels) and must operate according to the directing force or intelligence of its source of power.

Man has been deficient in understanding because his brain receiver did not vibrate to certain subtle influences. The dynamic cells in the gray matter of the nerves were not finely attuned and did not respond—hence sin, or falling short of understanding.

From the teachings of the Chemistry of Life we find that the basis of the brain or nerve fluid is a certain mineral salt known as potassium phosphate, or Kali Phos.

A deficiency in this brain constituent means "sin," or a falling short of judgment or proper comprehension. With the advent of the Aries Lord, God, or planet, cell-salts are rapidly coming to the fore as the basis of all healing. Kali phosphate is the greatest healing agent known to man, because it is the chemical base of material expression and understanding.

The cell-salts of the human organism are now being prepared for use, while poisonous drugs are being discarded everywhere. Kali phosphate is the especial birth salt for those born between March 21 and April 19.

These people are brain workers, earnest, executive and determined—thus do they rapidly use up the brain vitalizers.

The Aries gems are amethyst and diamond.

The astral colors are white and rose pink.

In Bible alchemy Aries represents Gad, the seventh son of Jacob, and means "armed and prepared"—thus it is said when in trouble or danger, "keep your head."

In the symbolism of the New Testament, Aries corresponds with the disciple Thomas. Aries people are natural doubters until they figure a thing out for themselves.

TAURUS—THE "WINGED BULL" OF THE ZODIAC

April 19 to May 20

* * *

The ancients were not "primitive men." There never was a first man, nor a primitive man. Man is an eternal verity—the Truth, and Truth never had a beginning.

The Winged Bull of Nineveh is a symbol of the great truth that substance is materialized air, and that all so-called solid substances may be resolved into air.

Taurus is an earth sign, but earth (soul) is precipitated aerial elements. This chemical fact was known to the scientists of the Taurian age (over 4000 years ago); therefore they carved the emblem of their Zodiacal sign with wings.

Those born between the dates, April 19th and May 20th, can descend very deep into materiality or soar "High as that Heaven where Taurus wheels," as written by Edwin Markham, who is a Taurus native.

What can be finer than the following from

this noted Taurian, he who has sprouted the wings of spiritual concept:

"It is a vision waiting and aware,
   And you must bring it down, oh, men of
      worth,
Bring down the New Republic hung in air
   And make for it foundations on the Earth."

Air is the "raw material" for blood, and when it is drawn in, or breathed in, rather, by the "Infinite Alchemist," to the blood vessels, it unites with the philosopher's stone, mineral salts, and in the human laboratory creates blood.

So, then, blood is the elixir of life, the "Ichor of the Gods."

The sulphate of sodium, known to druggists as Nat. Sulph., chemically corresponds to the physical and mental characteristics of those born in the Taurus month.

Taurus is represented by the cerebellum, or lower brain, and neck.

A deficiency in Nat. Sulph. in the blood is always manifested by pains in the back of head, sometimes extending down the spine, and then affecting the liver.

The first cell-salt to become deficient in symptoms of disease in the Taurus native is Nat. Sulph.

The chief office of Nat. Sulph. is to eliminate the excess of water from the body.

In hot weather the atmosphere becomes heavily laden with water and is thus breathed into the blood through the lungs.

One molecule of the Taurus salt has the chemical power to take up and carry out of the system two molecules of water.

Blood does not become overcharged with water from the water we drink, but from an atmosphere overcharged with aqueous vapor drawn from water in rivers, lakes or swamps, by heat of the sun above 70 degrees in shade.

The more surplus water there is to be thrown out of blood, the more sodium sulphate required.

All so-called bilious or malarial troubles are simply a chemical effect or action caused by deficient sulphate of soda.

Chills and fever are Nature's method of getting rid of surplus water by squeezing it out of the blood through violent muscular, nervous and vascular spasms.

No "shakes" or ague can occur if blood be properly balanced chemically.

Governing planet: Venus.

Gems: Moss-agate and emerald.

Astral colors: Red and lemon yellow.

In Bible Alchemy Taurus represents Asher, the eighth son of Jacob, and means blessedness or happiness.

In the symbolism of the New Testament, Taurus corresponds with the disciple Thaddeus, meaning firmness, or led by love.

THE CHEMISTRY OF GEMINI

May 20th to June 21st
* * *

One of the chief characteristics of the Gemini Native is expression. The cell-salt kali muriaticum (potassium chloride) is the mineral worker of blood that forms fibrine and properly diffuses it throughout the tissues of the body.

This salt must not be confused with the chlorate of potash, a poison (chemical formulae K. CLO_3).

The formulae of the chloride of potassium (kali mur) is K. Cl.

Kali mur molecules are the principal agents used in the chemistry of life to build fibrine into the human organism. The skin that covers the face contains the lines and angles that give expression and thus differentiate one person from another; therefore the maker of fibrine has been designated as the birth salt of the Gemini native.

In venous blood fibrine amounts to three in one thousand parts. When the molecules of kali mur falls below the standard, the blood fibrine thickens, causing what is known as pleurisy, pneumonia, catarrh, diphtheria, etc. When the circulation fails to throw out the thickened fibrine via the glands or mucus membrane, it may stop the action of the heart. Embolus is a Latin word meaning little lump, or balls; therefore to die of embolus, or "heart failure," generally means that the heart's action was stopped by little lumps of fibrine clogging the auricles and ventricles of the heart.

When the blood contains the proper amount of kali mur, fibrine is functional and the symptoms referred to above do not manifest. Gemini means twins. Gemini is the sign which governs the United States.

The astral colors of Gemini are red, white and blue. While those who made our first flag and chose the colors personally knew nothing of astrology, yet the Cosmic Law worked its will to give America the "red, white and blue."

Mercury is the governing planet of Gemini. The gems are beryl, aquamarine and dark blue stones. In Bible alchemy Gemini represents Issachar, the ninth son of Jacob, and means price, reward or recompense. In the symbolism, allegories of the New Testament, Gemini corresponds with the disciple Judas, which means service or necessity. The perverted ideas of an ignorant dark-age priesthood made "service and necessity" infamous by a literal rendering of the alchemical symbol, but during the present aquarian age, the Judas symbol will be understood and the disciple of "service" will no longer have to submit to "third degree methods."

> "Each life is fed
> From many a fountain-head,
> Tides that we never know
> Into our being flow,
> And rays from the remotest star
> Converge to made us what we are."

CANCER: THE CHEMISTRY OF THE "CRAB"

* * *

June 21 to July 22.

Cancer is the Mother Sign of the Zodiac.

The mother's breast is the soul's first home after taking on flesh and "rending the Veil of Isis."

The tenacity of those born between the dates, June 21 and July 22, in holding onto a home or dwelling place is well illustrated by the crab's grip, and, also, by the fact that it carries its house along wherever it goes in order that it may be sure of a dwelling.

The Angles (Angels) of the twelve Zodiacal Signs materialize their vitalities in the human microcosm. Through the operation of chemistry, energy creating, the intelligent molecules of Divine Substance make the "Word flesh."

The corner stone in the chemistry of the crab is the inorganic salt fluoride of lime, known in pharmacy language as Calcarea Flurica. It is a combination of fluorine and lime.

When this cell-salt is deficient in the blood, physical and mental disease (not-at-ease) is the result. Elastic fiber is formed by the union of the fluoride of lime with albuminoids, whether in the rubber tree or the human body. All relaxed conditions of tissue (varicose veins and kindred ailments) are due to a lack of sufficient amount of elastic fiber to "rubber" the tissue and hold it in place .

When elastic fiber is deficient in tissue of membrane between the upper and lower brain poles—cerebrum and cerebellum—there results a "sagging apart" of the positive and negative poles of the dynamo that runs the machinery of man.

An unfailing sign or symptom of this deficiency is a groundless fear of financial ruin.

While those born in any of the twelve signs may sometimes be deficient in Cal. Fluo., due to Mars or Mercury (or both) in Cancer at birth, Cancer people are more liable to symptoms, indicating a lack of this elastic fiber-builder than are those born in other signs.

Why should we search Latin and Greek lexicons to find a name for the result of a deficiency in some of the mineral constituents of blood? If we find a briar in our flesh, we say so in the plainest speech; we do not say, "I have got the briatitis or splintraligia."

When we know that a deficiency in the cell-salts of the blood causes the symptoms that medical ignorance has dignified and personified with names that nobody knows the meaning of, we will know how to scientifically heal by the unalterable law of the chemistry of life. When we learn the cause of disease, then, and not before, will we prevent disease.

Not through quarantine, nor disinfectants, nor "Boards of Health" will man reach the long sought plane of health; not through affirmations of health, nor denials of disease will bodily regeneration be wrought; not by dieting or fasting or "Fletcherizing" or suggesting, will the elixir of life and the philosopher's stone be found.

The "mercury of the sages" and the "Hidden manna" are not constituents of health foods.

Victims of salt baths and massage are bald before their time, and the alcohol, steam and Turkish bath fiends die young.

"Sic transit gloria mundi."

When a man's body is made chemically perfect, the operations of mind will perfectly express.

Gems belonging to the sign of the breast are black onyx and emerald; astral colors, green and russet, brown.

Cancer is represented by Zebulum, the tenth son of Jacob, and means dwelling place or habitation.

Matthew is the Cancer disciple.

LEO: THE HEART OF THE ZODIAC

July 22 to August 22
* * *

The Sun overflows with divine energy. It is the "brewpot" that forever filters and scatters the "Elixir of Life."

Those born while the Sun is passing through Leo, July 22 to August 22, receive the heart vibrations, or pulses, of the Grand Man, or

"Circle of Beasts." All the blood in the body passes through the heart and the Leo native is the recipient of every quality and possibility contained in the great "Alchemical Vase," the "Son of Heaven."

The impulsive traits of Leo people are symboled in the pulse which is a reflex of heart throbs.

The astronomer, by the unerring law of mathematics applied to space, proportion, and the so-far-discovered wheels and cogs of the uni-machine, can tell where a certain planet must be located before the telescope has verified the prediction. So the astro-bichemist knows there must of necessity be a blood mineral and tissue builder to correspond with the materialized angle (angel) of the circle of the Zodiac.

The phosphate of magnesia, in biochemic therapeutics, is the remedy for all spasmodic impulsive symptoms. This salt supplies the deficient worker or builder in such cases and thus restores normal conditions. A lack of muscular force, or nerve vigor, indicates a disturbance in the operation of the heart cell-salt, magnesia phosphate, which gives the "Lion's spring," or impulse, to the blood that throbs through the heart.

Leo is ruled by the Sun, and the children of that celestial sign are natural sun worshipers.

Gold must contain a small percent of alloy or base metal before it can be used commercially.

Likewise the "Gold of Ophir"—Sun's rays, or vibration—must contain a high potency of the earth salt, magnesia, in order to be available for use in bodily function. Thus through the chemical action of the inorganic (mineral and water) in the organic, Sun's rays and ether, does the volatile become fixed, and the word becomes flesh.

Leo people consume their birth salts more rapidly than they consume any of the other salts of the blood; hence are often deficient in magnesium. Crude magnesia is too coarse to enter the blood through the delicate mucus membrane absorbents, and must be prepared according to the biochemic method before taken to supply the blood.

Gems of Leo are ruby and diamond.

Astral colors, red and green.

The eleventh child of Jacob, Dinah, represents Leo and means judged. Simon is the Leo disciple.

VIRGO: THE VIRGIN MARY
* * *
August 22 to September 23

Virgin means pure. Mary, Marie, or Mare (Mar) means water. The letter M is simply the sign of Aquarius, "The Water Bearer."

Virgin Mary means pure sea, or water.

Jesus is derived from a Greek word, meaning fish. Out of the pure sea, or water, comes fish.

Out of woman's body comes the "word made flesh." All substance comes forth from air, which is a higher potency of water.

All substance is fish, or the substance of Jesus.

This substance is made to say, "Eat, this is My body; drink, this is My blood."

There is nothing from which flesh and blood can be made, but the one universal Air, Energy, or Spirit, in which man has his being.

All tangible elements are the effects of certain rates of motion of the intangible and unseen elements. Nitrogen gas is mineral in solution, or ultimate potency.

Oil is made by the union of the sulphate of potassium (potash), with albuminoids and aerial elements.

The first element that is disturbed in the organism of those born in the celestial sign Virgo is oil; this break in the function of oil shows a deficiency in potassium sulphate, known in pharmacy as kali sulph.

Virgo is represented in the human body by the stomach and bowels, the laboratory in which food is consumed as fuel to set free the minerals, in order that they may enter the blood through the mucous membrane absorbents.

The letter X in Hebrew is Samech or Stomach. X, or cross, means crucifixion, or change-transmutation.

Virgo people are discriminating, analytical and critical.

The microscope reveals the fact that when the body is in health little jets of steam are constantly escaping from the seven million pores of the skin. A deficiency in kali sulph. molecules causes the oil in the tissue to thicken and clog these safety valves of the human engine, thus turning heat and secretions back upon the inner organs, lungs, pleura, membrane of nasal passages, etc. And does it not seem strange that medical science, that boasts of such great progress, can invent no better term than "bad cold" for these chemical results?

Kali sulph. is found in considerable quantities in the scalp and hair. When this salt falls below the standard, dandruff or eruptions, secreting yellowish thin, oily matter or falling out of the hair, is the result.

Kali sulph. is a wonderful salt, and its operation in the divine laboratory of man's body, where it manufactures oil, is the miracle of the chemistry of life.

Governing planet, Mercury. Gems, pink jasper and hyacinth. Astral colors, gold and black.

In Bible alchemy Virgo is represented by Joseph, the twelfth son of Jacob, and means: To increase power, or "son of the right hand."

Virgo corresponds with the disciple Bartholomew.

LIBRA: THE LOINS

September 23-October 23
* * *

This alkaline cell-salt is made from bone ash or by neutralizing orthophosphoric acid with carbonate of sodium.

Libra is a Latin word, meaning scales or balance. Sodium, or natrum, phosphate holds the balance between acids and the normal fluids of the human body.

Acid is organic and can be chemically split into two or more elements, thus destroying the formula that makes the chemical rate of motion called acid.

A certain amount of acid is necessary, and is always present in the blood, nerve, stomach and liver fluids. The apparent excess of acid is nearly always due to a deficiency in the alkaline, Libra, salt.

Acid, in alchemical lore, is represented as Satan (saturn), while sodium phosphate symbols Christ (Venus). An absence of the Christ principle gives license to Satan to run riot in the Holy Temple. The advent of Christ drives the evil out with a whip of thongs. Reference to the temple in the figurative language of the Bible and New Testament always symbols the human organism. "Know ye not that your bodies are the Temple of the living God?"

Solomon's temple is an allegory of the physical body of man and woman. Soul-of-man's-temple—the house, church, Beth or temple made without sound of "saw or hammer."

Hate, envy, criticism, jealousy, competition, selfishness, war, suicide and murder are largely caused by acid conditions of the blood, producing changes by chemical poisons and irritation of the brain cells, the keys upon which Soul plays "Divine Harmonies" or plays "fantastic tricks before high heaven," according to the arrangement of chemical molecules in the wondrous laboratory of the soul.

Without a proper balance of the Venus salt, the agent of peace and love, man is fit for "treason, strategems and spoils."

The people of the world never needed the alkaline or Libra salt more than they do at the present time, while wars and rumors of wars strut upon the Stage of Life (1918).

The Sun enters Libra September 23 and remains until October 23.

Governing planet, Venus.

Gems, diamond and opal.

Astral colors are black, crimson and light blue.

Libra is an air sign.

In Bible alchemy, Libra represents Reuben, the first son of Jacob. Reuben means Vision of the Sun.

In the symbolism of the New Testament, Libra corresponds with the disciple Peter.

Peter is derived from Petra, a stone or mineral.

On thee, Peter (mineral), will I build my church, viz., beth, house, body or temple.

INFLUENCE OF SUN ON VIBRATION OF BLOOD AT BIRTH

Scorpio—October 24 to November 22

* * *

From Scorpion to "White Eagle" may seem a very long journey to one who has not learned the science of patience or realized that time is an illusion of physical sense.

The Zodiacal sign Scorpio is represented in human material organism by the sexual functions.

The esoteric meaning of sex is based in mathematics, the body being a mathematical fact. Sex in Sanscrit means Six.

"Six days of Creation" simply means that all creation, or formation, from self-existing substance, is by and through the operation of sex principle—the only principle.

Three means male, father, the spirit of the male, and son; this trinity forms or constitutes one pole of Being, Energy or Life—the positive pole.

The negative pole, female trinity; female spirit of mother and daughter.

Thus two threes or trinities produce six or sex, the operation of which is the cause of all manifestation. Those who understand fully realize the truth of the New Testament statement, "There is no other name under heaven whereby ye may be saved (materialized and sustained), except through Jesus Christ and Him Crucified." By tracing the words Jesus and Crucify (also Christ) to their roots a wonderful world of truth appears to the understanding.*

The possibilities of Scorpio people are boundless after they have passed through trials and tribulations, viz.: Crucifixion or crossification.

One of the cell-salts of the blood, calcarea, sulphate, is the mineral ("stone") that especially corresponds to the Scorpio nature. Crude Calcarea sulphate is gypsum or sulphate of lime.

While in crude form lime is of little value, but add water and thus transmute it by changing its chemical formation, and plaster of paris is formed, a substance useful and ornamental. Every person, born between October 24 and November 22, should well consider this wonderful alchemical operation of their esoteric stone and thus realize the possibilities in store for them on their journey to the "Eyrie of the White Eagle."

Scorpio people are natural magnetic healers, especially after having passed through the waters of adversity, as heat is caused by the union of water and lime.

---

*Explained in "Wonders of the Human Body."

Scorpio is a water sign, governed by Mars. Mars is "a doer of things," also fiery at times, therefore, it is well that the Scorpio native take heed lest he sometimes "boil over."

In Bible Alchemy, Scorpio is represented by Simeon, the second son of Jacob. Simeon means "hears and obeys." In the symbolism of the New Testament Scorpio corresponds with the disciple Andrew, to create or ascend.

The gems are topaz and malachite; astral colors, golden brown and black.

A break in the molecular chain of the Scorpio salt, caused by a deficiency of that material in the blood, is the primal cause of all the so-called diseases of these people. This disturbance, not only causes symptoms called disease in physical functions, but it disturbs the astral fluids and gray matter of brain cells and thereby changes the operation of mind into inharmony. Sin means to lack or fall short; thus chemical deficiencies in life's chemistry causes sin.

When man learns to supply his dynamo with the proper dynamics, he will "wash away his sins with the blood of Christ"—blood made with the "White Stone."

Calcium sulphate should not be taken internally in crude form; in order to be taken up by absorbents of mucus membrane the lime salt must be triturated, according to the Biochemic method, up to 3rd or 6th. By this method lime may be rendered as fine as the molecules contained in grain, fruit or vegetables.

Blood contains three forms of lime. Lime and fluorine for Cancer sign; lime and phosphorus for Capricorn sign, and lime and sulphur for Scorpio.

Lime should never be used internally below 3rd decimal trituration.

THE CHEMISTRY OF SAGITTARIUS

November 22-December 21

* * *

The mineral or cell-salt of the blood corresponding to Sagittarius is Silica.

Synonyms: Silicea, silici oxide, white pebble or common quartz. Chemical abbreviation, Si. Made by fusing crude silica with carbonate of soda; dissolve the residue, filter, and precipitate by hydrochloric acid.

This product must be triturated as per biochemic process before using internally.

This salt is the surgeon of the human organism. Silica is found in the hair, skin, nails, periosteum, the membrane covering and protecting the bone, the nerve sheath, called neurilemma, and a trace is found in bone tissue. The surgical qualities of silica lie in the fact that its particles are sharp cornered. A piece of quartz is a sample of the finer particles. Reduce silica to an impalpable powder and the microscope reveals the fact that the molecules

are still pointed and jagged like a large piece
of quartz rock. In all cases, where it becomes
necessary that decaying organic matter be dis-
charged from any part of the body by the process of suppuration, these sharp pointed particles are pushed forward by the marvelous intelligence that operates without ceasing, day
and night in the wondrous human Beth, and
like a lancet cuts a passage to the surface for
the discharge of pus. Nowhere in all the
records of physiology or biological research can
anything be found more wonderful than the
chemical and mechanical operation of this Divine artisan.

The bone covering is made strong and firm
by silica. In case of boils or carbuncle, the bio-
chemist loses no time searching for "anthrax
baccili" or germs, nor does he experiment with
imaginary germ-killing serum, but simply furnishes nature with tools with which the necessary work may be accomplished.

The Centaur of mythology is known in the
"Circles of Beasts that worship before the Lord
(Sun) day and night," as Sagittarius, the
Archer, with drawn bow. Arrow heads are
composed of flint, decarbonized white pebble or
quartz. Thus we see why silica is the special
birth salt of all born in the Sagittarius sign.
Silica gives the glossy finish to hair and nails.
A stalk of corn or straw of wheat, oats or bar-
ley would not stand upright except they contained this mineral.

Sagittarius people are generally swift and

strong; and they are prophetic—look deeply into the future and hit the mark like the archer. A noted astrologer once said: "Never lay a wager with one born with the Sun in Sagittarius or with Sagittarius rising in the east lest you lose your wealth."

The Sagittarius native is very successful in thought transference. He (or she) can concentrate on a brain, miles distant, and so vibrate the aerial wires that fill space that the molecular intelligence of those finely attuned to nature's harmonies may read the message.

Governing planet, Jupiter.

Gems, carbuncle, diamond and turquoise.

The astral colors are gold, red and green.

Sagittarius is a fire sign and is represented in Bible Alchemy by Levi, the third son of Jacob, meaning "joined or associated."

In the symbolism of New Testament Sagittarius corresponds with the disciple James, son of Alpheus.

The Chicago Evening Post, Wednesday, August 19, 1914, in commenting on "Signs of Wrath and Portents From the Heavens," says among other things: "And in England today are men with the modern scientific mind who say that we cannot disregard utterly the idea that the movements of the heavenly bodies have their effect upon men."

CAPRICORN: THE GOAT OF THE ZODIAC

December 21-January 19
* * *

Circle means Sacrifice, according to the Cabala, the straight line bending to form a circle.

Thus we find twelve Zodiacal signs sacrificing to the sun. Symbolized by the devotions and sacrifices of the twelve disciples to Jesus.

Twelve months sacrifice for a solar year.

Twelve functions of man's body sacrifice for the temple, Beth or "Church of God"—the human house of flesh.

Twelve minerals—known as cell-salts—sacrifice by operation and combining to build tissue.

The dynamic force of these vitalized workmen constitute the chemical affinities—the positive and negative poles of mineral expression.

The Cabalistic numerical value of the letters g, o, a, t, add up 12.

Very ancient allegories depict a goat bearing the sins of Israelites into the Wilderness.

In the secret mysteries of initiation into certain societies, the goat is the chief symbol.

In Alchemical lore the "Great Work" is commenced "in the Goat" and is finished in the "White Stone." Biochemistry is the "Stone the builders rejected" and furnishes the key to all the mysteries and occultism of the Allegorical Goat.

Those persons born between the dates December 21 and January 19 come under the influence of the Sun in Capricorn—the Goat. Capricorn represents the great business interests—trusts and syndicates—where many laborers are employed. Thus Capricorn symbols the foundation and frame-work of society—the commonwealth of human interests.

The bones of the human organism represent the foundation stones and framework of the soul's temple (soul of man's temple).

See Solomon's Temple. Bone tissue is composed principally of the phosphate of lime, known as calcarea phosphate or calcium phosphate. Without a proper amount of lime no bone can be formed, and bone is the foundation of the body.

A building must first have a foundation before the structure can be reared. Thus we see why the "Great Work" commences in the Goat. Lime is white—hence the "White Stone."

In the 2nd chapter and 17th verse of Revelation may be found the alchemical formula of the "White Stone."

"To him that overcometh will I give to eat of the hidden manna, and will give him a White Stone, and in the Stone a new name written which no man knoweth saving he that receiveth it."

In the mountains of India, it is said, a tribe dwells, the priests of which claim that man's complete history from birth to death is recorded in his bones. These people say the bones are secret archives, hence do not decay quickly as does flesh and blood.

When the molecules of lime phosphate fall below the standard, a disturbance often occurs in the bone tissue and the decay of bone, known as carries of bone, commences. Phosphate of lime is the worker in albumen. It carries it to bone and uses it as cement in the making of bone.

So-called Bright's disease (first discovered in a man named Bright) is simply an outflow of albumen via kidneys, due to a deficiency of phosphate of lime.

When the Goat Salt is deficient in the Gastric Juice and bile ferments arise from undigested foods, acids for which find their way to synovial fluids in the joints of legs or arms or hands and often cause severe pains, but why the chemical operation, which is perfectly natural, should be called rheumatism passeth understanding.

Non-functional albumen, caused by a lack of lime phosphate, is the cause of eruptions, abscesses, consumption, catarrh and many other so-called diseases.

But let us all remember that disease means not-at-ease, and that the words do not mean an entity of any kind, shape, size, weight or quality, but an effect caused by some deficiency of blood material, and that only.

Phosphate of lime should never be taken in crude form. It must be triturated to 6th x, according to the biochemic method, in milk sugar in order to be taken up by the mucous membrane absorbents, and thus carried into the circulation.

Capricorn people possess a deep interior nature in which they often dwell in the "Solitude of the Soul."

They scheme and plan and build air castles and really enjoy their ideal world. If they are sometimes talkative, their language seldom gives any hint of the wonderland of their imagination.

To that enchanted garden the sign, "No Thoroughfare," forever blocks the way.

The Capricorn gems are white Onyx and Moonstone. The astral colors are garnet, brown, silver-gray and black.

Capricorn is an earth sign.

In Bible alchemy, Capricorn represents Judah, the fourth son of Jacob, and means "the praise of the Lord." In the symbolism of the New Testament, Capricorn corresponds with the disciple John.

THE SIGN OF THE SON OF MAN: AQUARIUS

January 20 to February 19

* * *

O age of man: Aquarius,
 Transmuter of all things base,
"Son of Man in the Heavens,"
 With sun-illumined face."

Our journey was long and weary,
 With pain and sorrow and tears,
But now at rest in thy kingdom,
 We welcome the coming years.

Those born between the dates January 20 and February 19 are doubly blest, and babies to be born during that period for many years to come will be favored of the gods.

The Solar System has entered the "Sign of the Son of Man," Aquarius, where it will remain for over 2000 years. According to planetary revolutions the Sun passes through Aquarius once every solar year; thus we have the double influence of the Aquarius vibration from January 20 to February 19.

Air contains 78 per cent of nitrogen gas, believed by scientists to be mineral in ultimate potency. Minerals are formed by the precipitation of nitrogen gas. Differentiation is attained by the proportion of oxygen and aqueous vapor (hydrogen) that unites with nitrogen.

A combination of sodium and chlorine forms the mineral known as common salt. This mineral absorbs water. The circulation or distribution of water in the human organism is due to the chemical action of the molecules of sodium chloride.

Crude soda cannot be taken up by mucous membrane absorbents and carried into the circulation. The sodium molecules found in the blood have been received from vegetable tissue which drew these salts from the soil in high potency. The mineral, or cell-salts, can also be prepared (and are prepared) in biochemic or homeopathic potency as fine as the trituration of Nature's laboratory in the physiology of plant growth, and then they are thoroughly mixed with sugar of milk and pressed into tablets ready to be taken internally to supply deficiencies in the human organism. A lack of the proper amount of these basic mineral salts (twelve in number) are the cause of all so-called disease.

Common table salt does not enter the blood, being too coarse to enter the delicate tubes of mucous membrane absorbents, but this salt does distribute water along the intestinal tract.

Aquarius is known in astrological symbol as "The Water Bearer." Sodium chloride, known also as natrum muriaticum, is also a bearer of water, and chemically corresponds with the zodiacal angle of Aquarius.

The term angle, or angel, of the Sun may also be used, for the position of the Sun at birth largely controls the vibration of blood.

So, then, we have sodium chloride as the "birth salt" of Aquarius people.

The governing planets are Saturn and Uranus; the gems are sapphire, opal and turquoise; the astral colors are blue, pink and nile green. Aquarius is an air-sign.

In Bible Alchemy, Aquarius represents Dan, the fifth son of Jacob, and means "judgment," or "he that judges." In the symbolism of the New Testament, Aquarius corresponds with the disciple James.

Uranus, the revolutionary planet, known as the "Son of Heaven," is now in Aquarius, "Sign of the Son of Man," and will remain there until October, 1919.

PISCES: THE FISH THAT SWIM IN THE PURE SEA

February 19 to March 20

* * *

Most everybody knows that Pisces means fishes, but few there be who know the esoteric meaning of fish. Fish in Greek is Ichthus, which Greek scholars claim means "substance from the sea."

Jesus is derived from the Greek for fish; Mary, mare, means water; therefore we see

how the Virgin Mary, pure sea, gives birth to
Jesus, or fish. There are two things in the
universe—Jesus and the Virgin Mary—spirit
and substance. So much for the symbol or allegory.

From the earth viewpoint we say that the
Sun enters the Zodiacal sign Pisces February
19, and remains until March 21. This position
of the Sun at birth gives the native a kind,
loving nature, industrious, methodical, logical
and mathematical; sympathetic and kind to
people in distress.

In the alchemy of the Bible we find that the
sixth son of Jacob, Naphtali, which means
"wrestling of God," symbols Pisces, for the
Pisces natives worry and fret because they cannot do more for their friends or those in
trouble.

The phosphate of iron is one of the cell-salts
of human blood and tissue. This mineral has
an affinity for oxygen which is carried into the
circulation and diffused throughout the organism by the chemical force of this inorganic
salt. The feet are the foundation of the body.
Iron is the foundation of blood. Most diseases of Pisces people commence with symptoms indicating a deficiency of iron molecules
in the blood; hence it is inferred that those born
between the dates February 19 and March 21
use more iron than do those born in other
signs.

Iron is known as the magnetic mineral, due
to the fact that it attracts oxygen. Pisces peo-

ple possess great magnetic force in their hands and make the best magnetic healers.

Health depends upon a proper amount of iron phosphate molecules in the blood. When these oxygen carriers are deficient, the circulation is increased in order to conduct a sufficient amount of oxygen to the extremities—all parts of the body—with the diminished quantity of iron on hand. This increased motion of blood causes friction, the result of which is heat. Just why this heat is called fever is a conundrum; maybe because fever is from Latin fevre, "to boil out," but I fail to see any relevancy between a lack of phosphate of iron and "boiling out."

The phosphate of iron (ferrum phosphate), in order to be made available as a remedy for the blood, must be triturated according to the biochemic method with milk sugar up to the third or sixth potency in order that the mucus membrane absorbents may take it up and carry it into the blood. Iron in the crude state, like the tincture, does not enter the circulation, but passes off with the faeces and is often an injury to the intestinal mucous membrane.

The governing planet of this sign is Jupiter.

The gems are chrysolite, pink-shell and moonstone.

The astral colors are white, pink, emerald-green and black.

Pisces is a water sign.

In Bible alchemy, Pisces represents Naphtali, the sixth son of Jacob and means "wrestlings of God." In the symbolism of the New Testament, Pisces corresponds with the disciple Philip.

The birth of Benjamin is given in that wonderful allegory, the 35th chapter of Genesis.

Benjamin is therefore the 13th child of Jacob.

See article, "13, the Operation of Wisdom," page 81, Wonders of the Human Body.

> "The heavens declare the glory of God;
> And the firmament showeth his handiwork.
> Day unto day uttereth speech,
> And night unto night showeth knowledge.
> There is no language where
> There voice is not heard."

—Psalms, 19th Chapt., 1-5 V.

Made in United States
Orlando, FL
10 October 2023

37750048R00029